Colon Health

Second Edition
Revised and Updated

Louise Tenney, MH

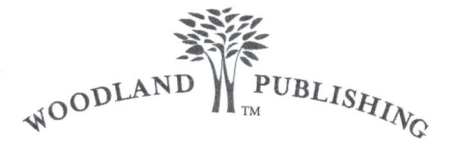

WOODLAND PUBLISHING

Copyright © 2007 Louise Tenney

All rights reserved. No part of this publication may be reproduced, stored in a retrieval system, or transmitted in any form without the prior written permission of the copyright owner.

For ordering information and bulk order discounts, contact:
Woodland Publishing, 448 East 800 North, Orem, UT 84097
Toll-free telephone: (800) 777-BOOK (2665)

Please visit our Web site: www.woodlandpublishing.com

Note: The information in this book is for educational purposes only and is not recommended as a means of diagnosing or treating an illness. All matters concerning physical and mental health should be supervised by a health practitioner knowledgeable in treating that particular condition. Neither the publisher nor the author directly or indirectly dispenses medical advice, nor do they prescribe any remedies or assume any responsibility for those who choose to treat themselves.

A cataloging-in-publication record for this book is available from the Library of Congress.

ISBN: 978-1-58054-435-1

Printed in the United States of America

Contents

Introduction 5

Digestion and Assimilation 6

Enzymes, Amino Acids, and Acidophilus 9

Constipation 11

Leaky Gut Syndrome 13

Parasites and Worms 16

Hiatal Hernia 18

Ileocecal Valve Syndrome 19

Allergies 21

Autointoxication 23

Candida 25

Cleansing for a Healthy Body 26

Conclusion 30

References 31

Introduction

As silly as it may sound, a healthy colon is the basis of a healthy body. In fact, most of us don't realize exactly how important a healthy colon is in maintaining optimal wellness.

Medical doctors used to focus on the health of the colon, but have actually regressed in recent years because of the rush to embrace the latest and greatest pharmaceutical remedy or diagnostic gadget. Modern medical doctors just aren't as good as they used to be in assessing what really causes disease: a unhealthy colon. Colon health should be a primary concern in the quest for a healthy body.

A healthy body naturally depends on the maintenance of a healthy digestive system. Food is the primary source of fuel for the body and if the wrong foods are eaten, the body will not function properly. Nutrients, vitamins, minerals, enzymes, amino acids, carbohydrates and lipids found in the foods we eat provide the energy and resources that quite literally keep us alive.

Unfortunately, the foods we eat are also addled with toxins and unnecessary substances that hinder our body's ability to remove waste properly. In addition, every drop of water, every breath of air, and every morsel of food we eat contains some toxic materials.

The body has its own natural means of dealing with the buildup of toxic materials. Acute diseases—colds, flus, etc.—are actually a cleansing process in the body. If the symptoms of acute diseases are suppressed with medications or other means, the toxins may not entirely be removed (which may be the precursor to a more serious condition in the future). Chronic conditions that develop may actually be a result of forbidding the body from ridding itself of toxic substances through acute disease.

In addition to acute disease, the body has another—and ultimately more important—way to "take the trash out." A healthy colon is the foundation of a healthy body, and learning natural methods to achieve colon health can be of utmost importance. Nutritious eating habits, cleansing diets, fiber sources, herbal remedies, and nutritional supplements can all contribute to total well-being. Above all, we must all understand that a healthy body absolutely requires a healthy colon.

Digestion and Assimilation

Ultimately, the food we eat determines exactly how efficiently all of our body's systems—and our body itself—works. Digestion is the body's first line of defense against foreign invaders that cause disease; in addition, the digestive system is also integral in supplying cells with much-needed nutrients and compounds.

Digestion, quite literally, is the breakdown of food throughout the gastrointestinal tract, the mouth, the stomach, the small and large intestines, and the colon. Digestion involves assimilation of nutrients (and toxins) by blood and lymph vessels, where they are transported to every cell for rebuilding, repair, and healing.

Along with nutrients, however, the blood and lymph vessels transport toxins to cells, where they are allowed to accumulate and cause cell degeneration and oxidation. As a result, the immune system is significantly weakened and resistance to disease vanishes. The body becomes sluggish and heavier; the skin becomes blotchy and the emotions unstable.

Causes of Digestive Problems

Many factors contribute to digestive disorders. These include:

- Alcohol
- Allergies
- Caffeine
- Candidiasis
- Cardiovascular diseases
- Colon congestion
- Constipation
- Enzyme deficiencies
- Gallbladder problems
- Hiatal hernia
- Hydrochloric acid deficiency
- Liver congestion
- Physiological imbalances
- Poor food combinations

- Sugar and sweets
- Tobacco
- Too little raw food
- Too much cooked food
- Ulcers
- White flour products

In a study conducted in the 1930s, Russian scientist Dr. Paul Kouchakoff discovered that the quantity of white blood cells in the intestines increases dramatically after cooked food is eaten. (Keep in mind that white blood cells are part of the immune system and always increase in number when there is a need to eliminate hostile invaders.) So apparently, a diet comprised primarily of cooked foods can initiate the beginnings of inflammation or disease. Cooked food places an added burden on the immune system and also contributes to digestive disturbances.

The same study found that eating raw foods did not increase white cell response. Even more remarkable, a Swiss nutritionist discovered that eating raw vegetables before eating cooked food prevented the increase of white blood cells in the intestines. (Clark, 56) For example, a salad with endive or watercress is very beneficial for digestion and will help heal and repair the stomach.

Unfortunately, we typically do the most harm to our health by what we eat and what we don't eat. In order to break down food, the stomach contains hydrochloric acid, which is powerful enough to dissolve metal. Hydrochloric acid also helps neutralize unwelcome substances and toxins that enter our bodies in the food we eat and the things we drink. But occasionally the stomach and its acid-based lines of defense break down, resulting in digestive malfunctions.

Nutrients for Proper Digestion

The following list summarizes the nutrients that the body needs in sufficient quantities for the gastrointestinal tract to properly digest food, assimilate essential nutrients, and adequately dispose of waste:

- Digestive enzymes are essential in the digestion of any food. Acidophilus is important for proper bowel function. Adequate amounts of acidophilus—a beneficial type of bacteria—help to keep pathogenic bacteria from growing in sufficient amounts to cause problems.

- Hydrochloric acid is needed for the assimilation of vitamins and minerals; especially vitamin C and calcium.

- B-complex vitamins help promote a healthy digestive tract. They assist enzymes in the metabolism of proteins, fats, and carbohydrates.

- Sodium is stored in the stomach wall and also in the joints. Sodium neutralizes acidity in the body, and is needed when there is a deficiency of hydrochloric acid.

- Calcium is essential to numerous metabolic processes. If the stomach lacks adequate amounts of hydrochloric acid, calcium and other essential minerals will not be sufficiently absorbed.

- Fiber is essential for proper digestion and elimination of food. Fiber reduces the absorption of fat, inhibits the absorption of undesirable estrogens (female hormones) into the bloodstream, and helps maintain a healthy, smooth-running digestive tract.

Herbal Aids for Proper Digestion

The following herbs can be very helpful in treating various digestive problems:

- Capsicum
- Garlic
- Gentian
- Ginger
- Goldenseal
- Licorice
- Papaya juice or tablets
- Psyllium powder

An herbal lower-bowel formula can stimulate daily bowel elimination and also clean the crust of waste that builds up on the colon walls. It's also important to avoid synthetic over-the-counter antacids. Natural remedies such as herbs, digestive enzymes, acidophilus and other beneficial probiotics, prebiotics (to encourage the growth of probiotics), and activated charcoal are readily available at your local health food store.

Enzymes, Amino Acids, and Acidophilus

Enzymes are essential for life—without them, our body's ability to ward off disease would be seriously limited. Enzymes act as catalysts—or "spark plugs"— that initiate and enable nearly every biochemical function in the human body. Enzymes help digest food, destroy parasites (worms, bacteria, etc.) and toxins that enter the body, and help neutralize damaging free radicals before they wreak havoc on cellular structures. Simply put, without enzymes, the body would fall apart. The lack of adequate enzymes in the standard American diet (SAD) as we approach the second decade of the twenty-first century is one reason why autoimmune diseases such as rheumatoid arthritis, chronic fatigue syndrome, fibromyalgia, and lupus have become so prevalent. Our bodies are just not getting adequate amounts of the enzymes they need to stay healthy and fight disease.

Amino Acids

For too long, nutrition researchers have turned a blind eye to the profound effects that amino acids have on our health. But today, scientists are recognizing the astonishing capabilities of amino acids in restoring and maintaining good health. In fact, amino acid therapy has proven to be useful in treating ailments as wide-ranging as:

- Alcoholism
- Anxiety
- Attention deficit disorder
- Autoimmune diseases
- Behavioral disorders
- Cancer
- Candidiasis
- Cardiovascular diseases
- Chronic fatigue syndrome
- Chronic pain
- Depression
- Diabetes
- Drug addiction
- Eating disorders
- Headaches
- Hypoglycemia
- Learning disorders
- Multiple chemical sensitivity
- Osteoarthritis
- Rheumatoid arthritis
- Reward deficiency syndrome
- Seizures

Most of the twenty-three identifiable amino acids can be manufactured by the body, but eight amino acids must be supplied in the diet. They are isoleucine, leucine, lysine, methionine, phenylalanine, theonine, tryptophan, and valine. Two more amino acids, cysteine and tyrosine, should also be classified as "essential" because they are derivatives of the essential amino acids methionine and phenylalanine.

In addition, two "nonessential" amino acids, histidine and arginine, should be considered "essential" for young children. Their bodies cannot meet the demands for histidine and arginine.

Acidophilus

The human body can be seen as a vast ecosystem that includes trillions of microorganisms. One of these microorganisms, *Lactobacillus acidophilus*, or acidophilus, is needed by the body for proper digestion and assimilation of nutrients. Amazingly, acidophilus has the ability to change and adapt to a myriad of environmental changes inside the intestines.

Acidophilus helps to protect the body from an overgrowth of the yeast *Candida albicans* and other microorgasnisms that invade and live in the body. *Lactobacillus acidophilus* actually adheres to the walls of the intestines and the vagina and prevents disease-causing microbes from taking hold. When the good acidophilus bacteria are compromised, there is suddenly room at the inn for the undesirable invading microbes, which quickly take root.

Acidophilus also consumes all the food reserves available to microorganisms; when invading bacteria encounter regions where acidophilus is plentiful, the bad bacteria simply pass through without taking up residence. Acidophilus is also responsible for producing acetic acids that lower the natural pH in the intestines, which discourages the growth of the other bacteria that flourish in a more acidic environment.

The intestinal and vaginal flora can be affected by various elements. The overuse of antibiotics, oral contraceptives, excessive sugar consumption, aspirin, antihistamines, cortisone, prednisone, coffee, and stress all contribute to an imbalance in the bacterial flora of the gastrointestinal tract. When the friendly bacteria are outnumbered, harmful substances may not be excreted from the body and can cause all sorts of problems.

Constipation

Constipation is a very serious health threat with far-reaching consequences. It is a common but dangerous ailment that afflicts every segment of our society. Bowel dysfunction can manifest itself in many ways, but the bottom line is that a clean and efficiently functioning colon is absolutely essential to our health, well-being, and longevity.

The current technical definition of constipation refers to a decrease in bowel movements or difficulty in the formation or passage of the stool. While this definition may be technically correct, it is incomplete and fails to explain all of the ramifications of a dysfunctional colon. In reality, several kinds of constipation exist, and most of us unknowingly suffer from one form or another. In his book *Colon Hygiene*, the famed natural health pioneer John Harvey Kellogg, MD, describes three forms of constipation:

Simple constipation: This condition arises when the elimination of the bowel content is not complete. Consequently, fecal matter remains in the bowels and gradually builds up and adheres to the colon wall. The condition can be the consequence of irregular eating schedules, overeating cooked food, a lack of exercise, and neglecting the urge to eliminate. This condition may signal the beginning of chronic constipation and may be a significant precursor to many of the ailments that plague humankind.

Cumulative constipation: The most common form of constipation, it is mostly confined to the lower part of the colon and is due to poor peristaltic action. The purpose of peristaltic waves—reflected in the urge to pass a bowel movement—is to propel the contents of the colon from the cecum to the rectum for eventual elimination. Lack of normal bowel action can cause injury to the colon walls and the ileocecal valve in the large intestine. As a result of cumulative constipation, straining is usually necessary to eliminate fecal matter from the body. This straining can eventually cause hemorrhoids (internal and external), varicose veins, lower back pain, and many other symptoms.

Latent constipation: this type of constipation typically occurs in people who suffer from chronic disease. Latent constipation takes years to develop, and most people are not aware of its presence because the bowels move regularly. Symptoms of this kind of constipation are numerous and include fatigue, headaches, bad breath, appendicitis, colitis, PMS, anxiety, and depression—and that is just the beginning of the list. (Kellogg, 195–200)

Diarrhea: It may seem strange that diarrhea is listed as a type of constipation, but the malady is caused by an irritation in the colon. Chronic diarrhea can occur when certain irritants adhere to the bowel walls and cannot be eliminated. The bowel reacts negatively and forces waste out as quickly as possible, resulting in diarrhea. Hardened bowel residue can be loosened and removed with herbal formulas.

Causes of Constipation

There are many causes of constipation, including:

- Aluminum-based antacids
- Antidepressants
- Anxiety
- Bowel adhesions
- Diabetes
- Drinking too little water
- Endocrine disorders
- Endometriosis
- Enlarged prostate
- Hemorrhoids
- Hydrochloric acid deficiency
- Ileocecal valve syndrome
- Iron supplements
- Lack of dietary fiber
- Lack of digestive enzymes
- Lack of exercise
- Narcotic pain killers
- Neurological disorders
- Physical obstruction
- Poor posture
- Pregnancy
- Slow transit time
- Stress
- Stretched colon from food overload
- Underactive thyroid gland
- Weak bowel muscles

Symptoms of Constipation

- Anxiety
- Bloating and gas
- Depression
- Development of hemorrhoids
- Incomplete bowel movements
- Indigestion

- Insomnia
- Painful bowel movements
- Sluggish feeling
- Tender or distended abdomen

Preventing Constipation

Adding fiber to the diet in combination with plenty of raw fruits and vegetables can work fabulously to prevent constipation. The amount of fiber recommended for anyone who suffers from constipation is 40 grams per day, which can be easily found in cereal sources of fiber combined with fruits and vegetables. Remember, however, that it is important to increase your water intake any time you increase your fiber consumption.

Leaky Gut Syndrome

Sherry A. Rogers, MD, describes leaky gut syndrome: "Leaky gut syndrome is a poorly recognized but extremely common problem that is seldom tested for. It represents a hyperpermeable intestinal lining. In other words, large spaces develop between the cells of the gut wall and bacteria, toxins and food leak in." (*Let's Live*, April 1995, 34–35)

If the lining of the intestinal tract becomes more permeable than normal, it can lead to serious health concerns. The large spaces that develop between the cells of the gut wall allow toxic material to enter the bloodstream. Under normal conditions these toxic substances will be eliminated, but when leaky gut syndrome occurs, parasites, bacteria, fungi, toxins, fats, and other foreign matter not normally absorbed enter the bloodstream. These microbes and other substances can put a strain on the liver's ability to detoxify the body.

When leaky gut syndrome causes antibodies to be released, they can attach to various body tissues leading to an inflammatory response. If the inflammation occurs in a joint, rheumatoid arthritis may result. If the antibodies attack the gut lining, various gastrointestinal problems can develop, such as Crohn's disease and colitis. Other related conditions include migraines, eczema, and a weakened immune response. The body's furious antibody response can produce leaky gut–like symptoms in just about any organ or area of the body.

Causes of Leaky Gut Syndrome

Leaky gut syndrome can be caused by a number of factors, including the standard American diet (SAD), other poor nutritional habits, lack of adequate fiber in the diet, and lack of adequate overall health care. Leaky gut syndrome manifests itself as an inflammation of the gut lining, which creates hyperpermeability that allows the contents of the colon to leak through the colon wall. Other causes of leaky gut syndrome include:

- Alcohol and caffeine
- Antibiotics
- Chemicals
- Enzyme deficiencies
- Molds and fungus
- Nausea after eating
- NSAIDs
- Parasite infections
- Poor diet

Symptoms of Leaky Gut Syndrome

- Abdominal distention
- Abdominal pain
- Aches and pains
- Chemical sensitivities
- Cognitive difficulties
- Diarrhea
- Difficulty exercising
- Fatigue
- Flu
- Food allergies
- Food sensitivities
- Frequent colds
- Fungal disease
- Infections
- Low-grade fever
- Memory deficit
- Nausea after eating
- Shortness of breath
- Skin rashes

Diseases Associated with Leaky Gut Syndrome

- Acne
- AIDS
- Asthma
- Autism
- Celiac disease
- Chemical sensitivities
- Chronic fatigue syndrome
- Cystic fibrosis
- Eczema
- Fibromyalgia
- Food allergies
- Food sensitivities
- Inflammatory bowel disease
- Liver disease
- Lupus
- Psoriasis
- Rheumatoid arthritis

Dietary Guidelines

- The following vegetable juice combinations will help eradicate leaky gut syndrome:
    - Carrot, celery, and endive
    - Carrot, parsley, and cabbage
    - Ginger, parsley, garlic, carrots, and celery

  Fasting on these juices two to three days a week will help speed healing of the digestive tract.

- Thermos-cooked grains help heal the digestive tract. They are rich in enzymes, vitamins, minerals, and protein. This slow-cooking process prevents destruction of the vital enzymes.

- Drink plenty of liquids, including pure water, electrolyte drinks without added sugar, fruit juices diluted with pure water, and almond milk, which is rich in calcium, magnesium, and protein. Almond milk can also be added to fruit drinks.

- Millet, buckwheat, and basmati rice can be eaten for breakfast. They are easy for the body to digest and are very nourishing.

- Raw fruits and vegetables, yams, avocados, and steamed vegetables all help to heal the digestive tract.

Nutritional Supplements
- Acidophilus
- Antioxidants
- B-complex vitamins
- Calcium and magnesium
- Essential fatty acids (flaxseed oil, fish oil, evening primrose oil)
- Plant digestive enzymes
- Vitamin A (beta carotene)
- Vitamin C with bioflavonoids

Herbal Aids
- Aloe vera juice
- Cat's claw
- Comfrey
- Goldenseal
- Grapeseed extract
- Licorice
- Pau d'arco

Parasites and Worms

Parasites and worms are scavengers and organisms that live within, upon, or at the expense of a host organism without contributing to the survival of the host. They can reside in the gastrointestinal tract and feed on toxins and waste material in the body. The most common types include roundworms (hookworms, pinworms, and threadworms) and tapeworms. The main problem with parasites is that they expel toxic and potentially deadly waste material into the host.

Parasites cause many diseases, including colon disorders, some types of cancer, chronic fatigue syndrome, and candidiasis. Usually inadequate sanitation is the cause of parasite infestations. If the body is free of toxins and an adequate amount of hydrochloric acid is being produced, parasites and worms and their larvae will be destroyed. However, a diet rich in carbohydrates, fats, and sugars provides the ideal food for parasites and worms in the body.

Worms and parasites can be contracted in may different ways. An individual may unknowingly come in contact with contaminated waste material. Walking barefoot on contaminated soil can lead to infestation. Ingestion of larvae or eggs from handling raw or partially cooked meat may also be the cause. Also, frequent use of antibiotics and other medications, a poor diet, and even stress can reduce beneficial intestinal flora and provide an environment for parasites and worms to thrive.

The microscopic parasite *Giardia lamblia*, which causes giardiasis, has been found in some municipal drinking water systems. It's most often found in streams and lakes, but it does sometimes enter our drinking water supplies. Animal waste is usually the source of giardia.

Too frequently, medical practitioners don't properly diagnose parasite infections, so if you have any of the symptoms listed below and you seek medical help, be sure to ask your health-care provider if you might have a parasite infection.

Symptoms of Parasitic Infection

- Abdominal pain
- Anemia
- Bloating and gas
- Colitis
- Colon disorders
- Constipation
- Diarrhea
- Fatigue
- Growth problems in children
- Headaches
- Ileocecal valve syndrome
- Loss of appetite
- Poor absorption of nutrients
- Rectal itching
- Weakened immune response
- Weight loss

Dietary Guidelines

- Eat a high-fiber diet full of raw vegetables, fruits, and whole grains.

- Pumpkin seeds, pomegranate seeds, sesame seeds, and figs can help rid the body of parasites and worms.

- Garlic, onions, cabbage, and carrots contain sulfur, which aids in expelling parasites from the body.

- Avoid sugar, refined foods, white flour products, chocolate, alcohol, tobacco, and caffeine.

- Strictly limit or eliminate meat and poultry, especially pork, from your diet. Always make sure that the meat is fully cooked.

- Adequate amounts of hydrochloric acid and digestive enzymes are very important. A healthy quantity of hydrochloric acid in the stomach creates an environment that is very hostile to any parasitic invaders.
- Blood, colon, and liver cleansers are necessary to get rid of the toxins that feed parasites and worms.

Nutritional Supplements

- Acidophilus
- B-complex vitamins
- Essential fatty acids
- Multivitamin/mineral supplement
- Vitamin C with bioflavonoids
- Zinc

Herbal Aids

- Aloe vera juice
- Black walnut
- Burdock
- Echinacea
- Garlic
- Goldenseal
- Grapeseed extract
- Pumpkin seed

Hiatal Hernia

The esophageal hiatus is a hole in the diaphragm that the esophagus passes through to join the top of the stomach. A hiatal hernia occurs when the stomach inches its way up through the hiatus and protrudes into the diaphragm (a hernia refers to any protrusion through connective tissue or the wall of a body cavity that is normally enclosed).

The major symptoms of hiatal hernia include heartburn, gastroesophageal reflux, and belching. Hiatal hernia is a common problem among the elderly, and it is estimated that up to 50 percent of the population over the age of forty suffers from some type this condition.

Symptoms of Hiatal Hernia

The principal symptoms of hiatal hernia are gastrointestinal reflux, chronic heartburn, and belching. Other symptoms include:

- Allergies
- Anxiety
- Bloating and gas
- Constipation
- Diarrhea
- Dizziness
- Fatigue
- Nausea
- Pressure below breastbone
- Regurgitation
- Vomiting

Dietary Guidelines

- Drink at least eight 8-ounce glasses of water a day.
- Eat several small meals a day in a calm environment and never eat within two hours of bedtime.
- Eat more whole grains.
- Eat more fruits and vegetables.
- Avoid meat.
- Avoid fat and fried foods.
- Avoid coffee, tea, alcohol, soda pop, and tobacco.

Nutritional Supplements

- Antioxidants
- B-complex vitamins
- Chlorophyll
- Coenzyme Q10
- Minerals
- Papaya juice or tablets
- Vitamin A (beta carotene)
- Vitamin C with bioflavonoids
- Zinc

Herbal Aids

- Aloe vera juice
- Gentian
- Ginger
- Goldenseal
- Marshmallow
- Slippery elm

Ileocecal Valve Syndrome

The ileocecal valve is made up of sphincter muscles that close the ileum (the point where the small intestine empties into the ascending colon, or jejunum). The ileocecal valve prevents toxins and other materials that are released by the appendix—which is close to the opening into the small intestine—from entering the small intestine.

In addition, the ileocecal valve helps to keep digested material in the small intestine until all nutrients have been absorbed. When the food residue is ready for elimination, the small intestine mixes it with mucus, bile, and other excretions and releases it systematically through the ileocecal valve into the large intestine. This prevents an overload of material for the body to eliminate.

Ileocecal valve syndrome occurs when toxic material from the colon is permitted to regurgitate back into the small intestine, where it is rapidly reabsorbed, leading to infection and disease.

Symptoms of Ileocecal Valve Syndrome

- Acne
- Constipation
- Diarrhea
- Duodenal ulcers
- Fatigue
- Irregular bowel movements
- Lower right bowel tenderness
- Migraine headaches
- Weakened immune response

Dietary Guidelines

- Eat a high-fiber diet, including whole grains. Soak the grains before cooking to avoid irritation.

- Avoid foods that cause constipation like dairy products, meat, and bananas.

- Eat stewed prunes, figs, and raisins for breakfast.

- Add more fresh fruits and vegetables to your diet. Use softer raw vegetables such as leaf lettuce, spinach, avocados, sprouts, and tomatoes at first.

- Reduce the amount of meat eaten.

- Take a fiber supplement to avoid constipation.

- Thermos-cooked grains are healing on the digestive tract. They are rich in enzymes, vitamins, minerals, and protein. This slow-cooking process protects the vital enzymes.

- Millet, buckwheat, and basmati rice can be eaten for breakfast. They are easy for the body to digest and very nourishing.
- Raw vegetables and fruits, steamed vegetables, yams, and avocados are all helpful in healing the digestive tract.

Nutritional Supplements

- Acidophilus
- Antioxidants
- B-complex vitamins
- Blue-green algae
- Calcium and magnesium
- Essential fatty acids
- Plant digestive enzymes
- Vitamin A (beta carotene)
- Vitamin C with bioflavonoids

Herbal Aids

- Aloe vera juice
- Cat's claw
- Comfrey
- Goldenseal
- Grapeseed extract
- Licorice
- Pau d'arco
- Slippery elm

Allergies

Allergies are the result of an immune system that is weakened by a poor diet, polluted air, chemicals, and other toxic substances. In addition, there are usually several reasons allergies develop. As a result, physicians have difficulty properly identifying what is causing the allergy and they end up only treating one allergy with drug therapy that masks the true problem.

Amazingly, the colon can help in the fight against allergies. Eating a lot of junk food, sugar, meat, and nutritionally poor food along with the toxins in the environment can cause the colon to become congested or constipated. When this constipation occurs, damaging chemicals and toxins reenter the bloodstream and force the immune system into action. Allergic substances, which are not as dangerous as the toxins and poisons we eat, are ignored by an immune system that is fighting off invasive compounds elsewhere in the body.

Symptoms of Allergies

- Arthritis
- Belching
- Bloating and gas
- Canker sores
- Colitis
- Constipation
- Diarrhea
- Eczema
- Gastroesophageal reflux
- Headaches
- Heartburn
- Hives
- Hyperactivity
- Indigestion
- Inflammation
- Irritability
- Itching
- Lethargy
- Nasal congestion
- Rashes
- Runny nose
- Sinusitis
- Sneezing
- Watery eyes

Dietary Guidelines to Prevent Allergies

- A cleansing diet can help to eliminate toxins from the blood.

- Digestive enzymes and hydrochloric acid can help with the digestion and absorption of food.

- Juice fasting with carrot, celery, and raw apple juice may be beneficial.

- Colon cleansing using gentle herbs can help with constipation.

- Keep your liver healthy by using a liver cleanse. The liver is responsible for ridding the body of accumulated toxins. It also helps to produce histamines, which protects the body against allergies.

- Avoid foods with additives. Stay away from FD&C yellow no. 5 dyes, along with BHA (butylated hydroxyanisole), BHT (butylated hydroxytouline), benzoates, annatto, eucalyptol, monosodium glutamate, and vanillin.

- Eliminate foods that cause allergies such as wheat, eggs, dairy products, caffeine, chocolate, shellfish, strawberries, tomatoes, and citrus fruits. After approximately four weeks of eliminating all of these foods, they can be reintroduced into the diet one at a time. Pay close attention to any recurrence of allergic symptoms. Stay away from foods that offer no nutritional value.

Nutritional Supplements

- Acidophilus
- B-complex vitamins
- Calcium and magnesium
- Coenzyme Q10
- Digestive enzyme combination
- Germanium
- Multivitamin/mineral supplement
- Potassium
- Tyrosine
- Vitamin A (beta carotene)
- Vitamin C with bioflavonoids

Herbal Aids

- Bee pollen
- Blessed thistle
- Burdock
- Echinacea
- Ephedra
- Garlic
- Goldenseal
- Kelp
- Lobelia
- Marshmallow
- Pleurisy root

Autointoxication

A healthy colon is essential for a healthy body. Autointoxication, toxemia, and constipation can lead to neurological disorders. Constipation may even be an underlying cause of some cases of depression, mood swings, stress, anxiety, insomnia, and even strokes.

In June 1917, an article entitled "Symptomatology of the Nervous System in Chronic Intestinal Toxemia" was read at the 68th Annual Session of the American Medical Association in New York City. It was written by G. Reese Satterlee, MD, and Watson W. Eldridge, MD, and it reported that 518 cases of neurological symptoms ranging from mild cognitive impairment to hallucinations were relieved by eliminating intestinal toxemia (Satterlee, 1414).

During periods of emotional distress, the stomach becomes irritated and it tightens up. Consequently, the blood supply is unable to reach the stomach lining and congestion and inflammation result. If this is allowed to continue, the cells of the stomach lining eventually die from lack of nourishment, setting the stage for a grim lineup of ailments: ulcers, colitis, appendicitis—and even cancer.

Constipation, which leads to a toxic colon, can overburden the liver. The liver is unable to filter out the increased amounts of toxins effectively, resulting in brain and nervous system disorders.

Dietary Guidelines

- Eat foods that offer nutritional support to the body.
- Add more raw fruits and vegetables and whole grains to the diet.
- Avoid foods that stress the body, such as alcohol, tobacco, caffeine, sugar, white flour, and other refined foods.

Nutritional Supplements

- Antioxidants
- B-complex vitamins with extra B6 and B12
- Calcium and magnesium
- Multivitamin/mineral supplement
- Vitamin C with bioflavonoids

Herbal Aids

- Bee pollen
- Black cohosh
- Burdock
- Ginger
- Ginkgo
- Ginseng
- Gotu kola
- Kava kava
- Lady's slipper
- Licorice
- Oatstraw
- Passionflower
- Prickly ash
- Skullcap
- Wood betony

Candida

Candida is a normally occurring fungus that lives in the mucous membranes, especially in the digestive tract and vagina. It can also be found in the sinuses, ear canals, and genitourinary tract. The body can handle normal amounts of this fungus, but in large amounts, it is detrimental to digestive health. Under normal conditions, candida lives in harmony with other organisms in the intestinal flora. Candidiasis (overgrowth of *Candida albicans*) is most common among women in their childbearing years, but it can also affect infants and children.

Problems arise when the body's natural immune function is compromised because of various conditions like a lack of sleep, poor diet, stress, drugs, antibiotics, birth control pills, lack of exercise, and environmental pollutants. Anything that weakens the immune system will in turn encourage the growth of candida. A strong, healthy immune system will contain relatively small amounts of candida, but when the immune system falters candida can rapidly take hold.

Symptoms of Candidiasis

- Bad breath
- Chronic infections
- Constipation
- Depression
- Digestive disorders
- Fatigue
- Feeling spaced out
- Indigestion
- Migraine headaches
- Panic attacks
- Sore throat
- Swollen glands
- Thyroid problems

Dietary Guidelines

- Eliminate sugar, honey, white flour products, yeast breads, wine, beer, fruit juices, cheese, mushrooms, junk food, refined foods, and vinegar products from the diet.

- Eat only small amounts of fruit until the yeast is under control.

- Millet, brown rice, and other whole grains are a good choice.

- Eat a lot of raw and steamed vegetables.
- Beans are a good source of protein.
- Almonds and nuts are good, but avoid peanuts.
- A great drink can be made from carrots, parsley, garlic and ginger.
- Add fiber to the diet—it helps to cleanse the colon and eliminate toxins.

Nutritional Supplements

- Acidophilus
- B-complex vitamins
- Blue-green algae
- Caprylic acid
- Coenzyme Q10
- Digestive enzyme combination
- Multivitamin/mineral supplement
- Olive oil
- Vitamin A (beta carotene)
- Vitamin C with bioflavonoids
- Vitamin E

Herbal Aids

- Barberry
- Cat's claw
- Dong quai
- Echinacea
- Garlic
- Pau d'arco

Cleansing for a Healthy Body

In order to make health a way of life, eating patterns need to be changed. Restoring health to the body is impossible without cleansing the colon, blood, and lymphatic systems. Poor eating habits are the main reason the body is laden with toxins and poisons. The body can heal itself, but a cleansing and eliminating program is necessary to retain health and in allowing the body to heal.

Suggested Transition Diet

Before breakfast you can take supplements that for whatever condition you have. If you have candida, for example, take acidophilus first thing in the morning on an empty stomach, and use appropriate nutrients, foods, and herbs that support the elimination of candida. If you have hypoglycemia, eat the appropriate diet, supplements, and herbs to strengthen the body to overcome this condition.

Breakfast should consist of fruits such as cantaloupe, watermelon, peaches, grapes, pears, apricots, apples, and citrus fruit. An hour after eating the fruit, have a protein drink or eat some Thermos cereal, millet, or a brown rice dish. You can also drink fresh fruit and vegetable juices; they should always be diluted with half pure water.

Lunch can consist of salads using sprouts of all kinds, grain soups, steamed and raw vegetables. Use brown rice and millet dishes. You can also drink fresh tomato vegetable cocktail juices.

Dinner should be lighter than breakfast and lunch. You can drink fresh vegetable juices, steamed vegetables, baked potatoes, brown rice and millet dishes along with fresh salads.

Cleansing Diet (from the Seneca Indians)

The reason this diet is beneficial is the first day the colon is cleansed, and the second day toxins are released. Salt and excessive calcium deposits in the muscles, tissues, and organs are eliminated. On the third day, the digestive tract is supplied with healthy mineral-rich bulk. On the fourth day blood, lymph, and organs are cleansed.

First Day: Eat fruit, all you want, such as apples, berries, watermelon, pears, cherries, and apricots, but no bananas.

Second Day: Drink all the herb tea you want, such as chamomile, raspberry, spearmint, hyssop, pau d'arco, and red clover blends. If you sweeten the tea, use pure maple syrup.

Third Day: Eat all the vegetables you want; eat them raw, steamed, or both.

Fourth Day: Make a pan of vegetable broth using cauliflower, cabbage, onion, green pepper, parsley, or whatever you have on hand. Season with natural salt or vegetable seasoning. Drink only the rich mineral broth all day.

Cleansing the Liver

- Take a hydrochloric acid formula before meals.
- Take plant digestive enzymes during or after meals.
- Goats whey powder is rich in minerals, especially natural

sodium, which will help heal and repair the digestive tract. Use a tablespoon three times a day.
- Take a combination digestive herb supplement. Herbal formulas will supply nutrients to help stimulate and increase enzyme activity.
- Use an herbal lower bowel formula to cleanse the colon.
- Take an herbal supplement to help strengthen and repair the liver.
- Main herbs include gentian, licorice, goldenseal, fennel, blue-green algae, barley grass, catnip, and alfalfa.
- Assisting herbs include Oregon grape, milk thistle, dandlion, barberry, cruciferous vegetables, and barberry.
- Transporting herbs include capsicum, ginger, turmeric, lobelia, aloe vera, papaya, and peppermint.

Cleansing the Kidneys

- Minerals will help restore health to the kidneys.
- A potassium formula and goat's whey powder will heal the entire digestive tract as well as the kidneys.
- Take an herbal kidney cleansing and strengthening formula.
- Main herbs include oatstraw, cornsilk, uva ursi, goldenseal, pau d'arco, dandelion, horsetail, juniper, cranberry powder, and watermelon seeds. Assisting herbs include: marshmallow, kelp, comfrey, echinacea, mullein, and slippery elm.
- Transporting herbs include lobelia, ginger, peppermint, prickly ash, and capsicum.
- Acidophilus helps prevent infections and increases friendly bacteria.
- Chlorophyll and blue-green algae clean and heal infections and blood.

Cleansing the Colon

- Proper digestion will help speed the colon cleanse.
- An herbal cleansing tea is one way to get started on a colon cleanse.
- An herbal fiber formula is essential.
- A lower bowel cleanser is very important to help clean and loosen encrusted material on the colon walls.

- Main herbs are cascara sagrada, butternut bark, rhubarb, and burdock.
- Assisting herbs include fenugreek, slipper elm, licorice, kelp, Irish moss, blue green algae or other chlorophyll sources, or goldenseal.
- Transporting herbs are lobelia, capsicum, fennel, ginger, and peppermint.
- The following herbs should be used to rebuild and strengthen the colon walls: bee pollen, kelp, blue green algae, slippery elm, comfrey, marshmallow, aloe vera juice, and papaya.

Cleansing the Lungs

- Follow guidelines for digestion, liver and colon cleansing.
- Take a formula for cleansing and strengthening the lungs.
- Main herbs include ephedra, fenugreek, mullein, marshmallow, boneset, echinacea, chlorophyll and other green sources, and elecampane.
- Assisting herbs are: myrrh, licorice, pleurisy, hops, skullcap, comfrey, plantain, and eucalyptus.
- Transporting herbs are lobelia, capsicum, ginger, prickly ash.

Cleansing the Skin

- Colon, liver, kidney and blood cleansers are needed when cleansing the skin.
- Skin brushing will help speed the cleansing of the skin. Use natural cleansers for the skin to prevent clogging up the pores and preventing skin elimination.
- Faulty fat metabolism is a cause of most skin diseases. Foods rich in omega-3 and gamma-linoleic acids will help remedy this problem.
- Herbal formulas for the cleansing the skin can help.
- Main herbs are red clover, yellow dock, sarsparilla, burdock, yarrow, alfalfa, kelp, marshmallow, and sassafras.
- Assisting herbs include chlorophyll sources, rose hips, fenugreek, licorice, and thyme.
- Transporting herbs are ginger, cloves, fennel, lobelia, cayenne, and rosemary.

Cleansing the Blood and Lymphatics
- Eat healthy foods.
- Hydrochloric acid and digestive enzymes improve and repair the digestive system.
- Occasional fasting is necessary to help the body heal itself.
- Use an herbal formula to help cleanse the blood.
- Main herbs are red clover, pau d'arco, chapparal, echinacea, burdock, Oregon grape, goldenseal, ho shou wu, milk thistle, and suma.
- Assisting herbs are sheep sorrel, peach bark, licorice, astragalus, hyssop, myrrh gum, sarsaparilla, dandelion, wild yam, yellow dock, and cat's claw.
- Transporting herbs include prickly ash, ginger, lobelia, capsicum, kelp, fennel, cinnamon, and peppermint.

Cleansing the Body of Parasites and Worms
- Hydrochloric acid and digestive enzymes are very important.
- Blood, colon, and liver cleansers are necessary to get rid of the toxins that parasites and worms feed on.
- Eliminate white flour and sugar products. Eat a diet using fresh and steamed vegetables. Salads are important but need to be rinsed in apple cider vinegar to kill the larva.
- Take an herbal formula to destroy and expel worms from the body.
- Main herbs are black walnut hulls, wormwood, garlic, cloves, chaparral, gentian, pumpkin seeds, tea tree oil, cascara sagrada, aloe vera, and licorice.
- Assisting herbs are rhubarb, barberry, gentian, blue green algae, thyme, calendula, and alfalfa.
- Transporting herbs include lobelia, ginger, prickly ash, peppermint, and capsicum.

Conclusion

As more individuals become aware of their nutritional deficiencies, natural approaches to replenishing the body are being sought. The digestive system has often been overlooked as a factor in overall body health. If food and supplements are not absorbed and assimilated, the nutrients may not reach the bloodstream to nourish the entire body.

Colon health is more important than most people realize. The digestive process is directly related to the health of the body, the immune system, and even longevity. When any disease occurs, it is basic to look to the colon first for treatment. Following the example of doctors from the past may assist in promoting future health.

Start by understanding what it means to have a healthy colon. Gradually add fiber, nutritional supplements, and herbal helps along with a change in diet. Slowly change eating habits. It does not have to happen overnight. Eliminate unhealthy, nutrition robbing foods from the diet. Stress whole grain foods, fruits and vegetables.

We all need to take a look at our lifestyle habits and examine areas that need improvement. Most of us can certainly improve on the food we eat and feed our families. Small changes may mean significant improvement in health. Taking action now may mean a longer, healthier and happier life.

Bibliography

Balch, James F., MD, and Phyllis A. Balch, *Prescription for Nutritional Healing* (Garden City Park, NY: Avery Publishing Group, 1997).

Bateson-Koch, Carolee, *Allergies, Disease in Disguise* (Burnaby, BC Canada: Alive Books, 1994).

Brown, Donald J. *Herbal Prescription for Better Health* (Rocklin, CA: Prima Publishing, 1996).

Castleman, Michael, *Nature's Cures* (Emmaus, Pennsylvania: Rodale Press, Inc., 1996), 176.

Challem, Jack, "Good Bacteria that Fight the Bad," *Let's Live*, October, 1996, 55.

Chichoke, Anthony J., *Enzymes and Enzyme Therapy* (New Cannan, Connecticut: Keats Publishing, 1994).

Christopher, John R., *Regenerative Diet* (Springville, UT: Christopher Publications, 1982).

Clark, Linda, T*he New Way to Eat* (Millbrae, CA: Celestial Arts, 1980).

Cohen, M.L. "Epidemiology of drug resistance: implications for a post-antimicrobial era," *Science*, (1992;257) 1050–1055.

Elkins, Rita. *The Complete Fiber Book* (Pleasant Grove, UT: Woodland Publishing, Inc., 1996).

Elkins, Rita, *The Complete Home Health Advisor* (Pleasant Grove, UT: Woodland Publishing, Inc., 1994).

Fitch, William E. MD, "Putrefactive Intestinal Toxemia," *Medical Journal and Record* (132) (August 20, 1930): 189.

Galland, Leo, MD, *Superimmunity for Kids* (NY: Copestone Press, Inc., 1988).
Hawley, Clark W., MD, "Autointoxication and Eye Diseases," *Ophthalmology Magazine* 10 (14) (194): 663–74).
Hobbs, Christopher, *Foundations of Health* (Capitola, CA: Botanica Press, 1992).
Jensen, Bernard, *Tissue Cleansing Through Bowel Management* (Escondido, CA: Bernard Jensen Enterprises, 1993).
Keji, C. and S. Jun, "Progress of research of ischemic stroke treated with Chinese medicine," *Journal of Traditional Chinese Medicine.* (12) (1992): 204–10.
Kellogg, John Harvey, MD, *Colon Hygiene* (Good Health Publishing Co., 1916).
Kritchevsk, David, Charles Bonfield and James W. Anderson, Eds., *Dietary Fiber.* (New York: Plenum Press, 1988, 140).
Lane, Sir. W. Arbuthnot, MD, *The Prevention of the Diseases Peculiar to Civilization* (NY: Foundation for Alternative Cancer Therapies, revised 1998).
Livingston-Wheeler, Virginia, MD, *The Conquest of Cancer* (NY: Franklin Watts, 1984).
Michnovicz, Jon J., *How to Reduce Your Risk of Breast Cancer* (NY: Warner Books, 1994).
Monte, Tom, *World Medicine, The East-West Guide to Healing Your Body* (NY: Putnam Publishing Group, 1993).
Rogers, Sherry A., MD, *Let's Live,* April 1995, 34–35.
Rogers, Sherry A, MD, *Wellness Against All Odds* (Syracuse, NY: Prestige Publishing, 1994).
Satterlee, Reese, MD, and Watson W. Eldridge, MD, "Symptomatology of the Nervous System in Chronic Intestinal Toxemia," *Journal of the American Medical Association* 69 (17) (1917): 1414.
Scheer, James F., "Acidophilus, Nature's Antibiotic," *Better Nutrition for Today's Living,* August, 1993, 34.
Simone, Charles B., MD, *Cancer and Nutrition* (Garden City Park, NY: Avery Publishing, 1992).
Somer, Elizabeth, *Nutrition for Women, The Complete Guide.* (New York: Henry Holt and Company, 1993) 382–84.
Story J.A., "Dietary fiber and lipid metabolism," *Medical Aspects of Dietary Fiber,* (New York: Plenum Medical, 1980, 138).
Stuck, J.M., MD, *Intestinal Toxemia in Diagnosis and Treatment* (NY: A.R. Elliot Publishing Co., 1932).
Tenney, Louise, *Encyclopedia of Natural Remedies* (Pleasant Grove, UT: Woodland Publishing, Inc., 1995).
Tenney, Louise, *The Natural Guide to Colon Health* (Pleasant Grove, UT: Woodland Publishing, Inc., 1997).
Tenney, Louise, *Today's Herbal Health for Women* (Pleasant Grove, UT: Woodland Publishing, Inc., 1996).
Tenney, Louise, *Today's Herbal Health* (Pleasant Grove, UT: Woodland Publishing, Inc., 2006).
Tenney, Louise, *Nutritional Guide* (Pleasant Grove, UT: Woodland Publishing, Inc., 1994).
Vogel, A. MD, "Improved Liver Function," *Bestways,* Sept. 1986, 31.
Willet, et al, "Relation of meat, fat and fiber intake to the risk of colon cancer in prospective study among women." *New England Journal of Medicine* (23): 1664–72.